Listening to Babies

Empathic Guide for Craniosacral Practitioners

Richard Kramer BSc RCST

Copyright © 2022 Richard Kramer All rights reserved

The characters and events portrayed in this book are true but names have been changed.
No part of this book may be reproduced, or stored in a retrieval system, or transmitted in any form or by any means, electronic, mechanical, photocopying, recording, or otherwise, without express written permission of the publisher.

ISBN: 9798837300714

Cover design: Richard Kramer
Models: Baby Lola and Zoe
Photography: Alesio Tatore & Richard Kramer

Library of Congress Control Number: 2018675309
Printed in the United States of America

Acknowledgments:

I want to give my heartfelt gratitude to my partner Deborah, who has inspired me with her valuable suggestions over the many months of this creation.
My blessings go out to Jude for her infinite patience, wisdom and performing the very arduous task of editing.
I also want to convey my love and appreciation to my children, Josh and Hannah, who encouraged me to create this book.

At the still point of the turning world.
Neither flesh nor fleshless;
Neither from nor towards;
at the still point, there the dance is.

from T.S.Eliot 'Burnt Norton' , Four Quartets 1935

Contents:

Part 1: Introduction   Page 5

Part 2: Baby Trauma   Page 11

Part 3: Case History   Page 18

Part 4: Continuing the Enquiry   Page 23

Part 5: Fish, Babies, and the Polyvagal System
                                              Page 32

Part 6: Empathy, Love and Attachment theory
                                              Page 38

Part 7: Stillness   Page 50

Part 8: Feeding & Tongue-Tie   Page 56

Part 9: New Parents Look After Yourselves
                                              Page 61

Part 10: Giving & Receiving from the Community
                                              Page 66

Part 1: Introduction

Craniosacral therapy is highly successful in supporting babies in their recovery from birth trauma and associated conditions. But craniosacral practitioners starting their practices often feel cautious working with babies. Why?

Clearly, there is a demand to work with babies, as parents and carers hear from others how useful it has been.

It is often sought out because conventional medicine doesn't offer a holistic approach and may fail to fully appreciate the impact birth trauma can have on a neonate in their first weeks of life.

Providing craniosacral therapy for babies soon after birth could offer generations to come a good start in life, experiencing calm and easy adjustment to the world around them. Furthermore, it could reduce the numbers of anxious parents filling GP surgeries and be cost effective to the NHS.

Craniosacral therapy offers a non-invasive solution and consequently there is a place for this therapy for babies – so why the reluctance by practitioners?

Training colleges generally discourage newly qualified craniosacral therapists from initially working with babies. This is because it takes time and experience for new graduates in this field to be fully aware of their own 'internal' environment and state of grounding. Anything less could potentially retrigger a baby's trauma.

Furthermore, working with babies is a specialised area and requires advanced postgraduate training. Babies are not like adults, they need extra-careful handling, they do not remain still, they often cry and may be wary of being treated, they quickly become bored and need entertaining! In addition, they can't say where they feel discomfort or provide verbal feedback as such, and add to this mix, anxious parents may want quick results!

Such constraints, result in fewer practitioners working in this field. However, for the many babies who have received craniosacral therapy, it is highly successful in supporting them in their recovery from birth trauma and associated conditions.

But why is craniosacral therapy successful? This is a valid question asked by new graduates in this field.

Furthermore, my experience with babies doesn't fit neatly into the professional training I had received, nor anything that could be found in the literature at the time.

Craniosacral training develops a heightened sensitivity to the body's anatomy, fluid movements, fascial tissue twists and tensions, bony misalignments and lesions, internal rhythms, and so on.

All these can be palpated by an experienced practitioner with the subject lying still. But as we know, babies generally do not lie still – wriggling, and continuously thrashing their arms and legs here and there. Under these circumstances it is nigh on impossible to feel any subtle fluid or energy shifts, tissue reorganisation, etc.

In recent years there has been increased development in our understanding of the physiology and biochemistry of fluid movement and kinetics in and around the central and autonomic nervous systems, and interesting techniques have emerged from these concepts.

Despite increased understanding this does not offer, as such, a model of working with babies.

Consequently, it is no coincidence that in standard craniosacral textbooks there is little or no guidance to new practitioners, who wish to work with babies, other than what is essentially an osteopathic approach of palpating for bone and tissue lesions.

However, my experience has shown that approaching babies sensitively, as outlined here has led to good outcomes.

To understand why babies respond well to this therapy a different model is required that involves listening, observation and careful, detailed collation of a case history, not only of the baby's experience but of the mother before and during her pregnancy, plus her and her partner's birth history.

An awareness of the prevailing family dynamics can be added to this mix. All these factors could be in the baby's psyche as historical experiences and memories.

To arrive at a working model perhaps the question to ask should be,

'How do we therapeutically approach a baby'?

Underlying this must be the significant understanding that babies are sentient beings. 'Sentient' means having the ability to be aware of sensations and feelings. Babies can perceive and express emotions including anger, fear, contentment, and love. Many others have expressed the same. [1]

The emphasis outlined in this book will be to approach a baby from the baby's 'own experience', their trauma, their emotional state, and their needs.

Consequently, this translates into a model for the craniosacral therapist to engage with the baby's experience from prenatal to postpartum.

The basic understanding will be that the baby has faced trauma to varying degrees and needs support in processing this experience.

---

[1] See Association for Prenatal and Perinatal Psychology and Health for many publications on this topic. https://birthpsychology.com/

It should also be said that the mother also has experienced strong emotions throughout, from the time of her pregnancy onwards. She may have experienced shock, terror perhaps, tissue trauma, sadness, happiness - in fact the whole gamut of feelings. But emotionally for her there is a huge difference compared to her baby, because she has the capacity to rationalise and process the events, such as:

'I felt I wasn't ready'

'What went wrong?'

'Could this have been predicted?

'What went well?' '

Could it have been any different?'

A baby experiences trauma but cannot rationalise this. The impact of the pregnancy and birth must be 'processed' to move on, and babies need help to achieve this.

They can overcome the trauma to a large extent given time, but with craniosacral therapy this period is significantly reduced, sometimes with immediate effect.

This is the main reason craniosacral therapy is successful with babies, as it offers a relatively quick respite for the baby from their 'internal' terrors.

The approach expressed here will be practical and baby centric. However, the ideas presented are not new or unique but are applied with sensitivity that is associated with this therapy, offering respect, appreciation, understanding and love for the baby.

Taking this clinical path is adventurous and rewarding, as craniosacral therapy can make a significant difference to babies' lives and those around them.

◆◆◆

Part 2: Baby Trauma

How would you recognise a traumatised baby?

The following list of clues to assist in recognising trauma is not exhaustive. Perhaps only one or two characteristics will be initially apparent:

1. The baby will be a poor sleeper; being in an almost constant state of arousal and hypervigilance.

2. Hypervigilant babies may sleep for limited periods only, possibly waking and crying every hour or so. Sleeping will be light.

3. The baby will be easily startled, displaying the Moro response. Even when falling asleep they may self-startle themselves awake [2]

4. Generally unhappy and clingy. Wanting the touch of their parent. This can range from intermittently to most of the time.

---

[2] The Moro reflex refers to an involuntary motor response involving the infant suddenly splaying their arms and moving their legs before bringing their arms in front of their body.
https://en.wikipedia.org/wiki/Moro_reflex

5. Reluctance to orientate to visual or auditory stimuli except from the parent.

6. Needing to comfort feed, which may be very often and short in duration.

7. Poor eye contact. Can easily become overwhelmed if stared at by anyone other than the parent.

8. Inconsolable crying, a feature also associated with colic.

9. Colic can be a consequence of trauma, displaying many of these symptoms.

10. Weak grasp, due to not engaging fully with the world around them.

One may think a baby's case history would clearly suggest any existence of trauma, but this isn't always the case. Sometimes it isn't obvious what has contributed to a traumatic state. Even when the pregnancy and birth seemed to have proceeded without difficulty, baby trauma may arise for some unknown reason.

Conditions arising from trauma:

1. **Eczema:**
Its appearance may be delayed as it can arise from anxiety and stress.

2. **Colic:**
A wide spectrum condition, which is quite unpredictable in its severity. Can arise from a palpable compaction of the upper body and cranium. The strong uterine contractions

may have contributed to this condition, which can also compromise dorsal vagal activity on the gut throughout its length.

Features of colic include inconsolable crying for several hours especially in the early evening. In addition, abdominal discomfort will be present affecting mainly the stomach and small intestine. This does not explain why colic is found with caesarean babies, who generally have not experienced uterine contractions. It is possible under these circumstances that the sudden and dramatic shock of their exit from the uterus, or other uterine trauma gives rise to a similar contraction by the body and disturbance of the vagus.

3. **Oesophageal gastric reflux:**
Often resulting from an immature oesophageal sphincter, but also may be on the same spectrum as colic, with vagal dysfunction.

There is the characteristic arching of the baby's back accompanied by screaming and crying. Very often there is a dislike of baby car-seats, as this puts further pressure on the abdomen.

Parents find it helpful to keep their baby upright while feeding and carrying. The baby may experience considerable discomfort with this condition as the stomach acid rises in the oesophagus.

4. **'Silent reflux':**
This presents with little or no crying, is less obvious but characterised by the baby appearing to be tasting lemon

juice for the first time, as gastric juice in small quantities enters the mouth.

It must be assumed there will always be an element of trauma in a neonate, no matter the nature of the birth whether vaginal or caesarean.

There is a further dimension contributing to trauma - babies can experience trauma based predominately on fear as the following account suggests.

Case History: Baby Johnny

Kate, the mother of Johnny, reported the pregnancy was a frightening time. She had been trying to get pregnant for several years. Both partners were found to be in good health and there were no obvious reasons to suggest why pregnancy couldn't occur. As she was reaching her late-30s she sought in-vitro fertilisation which eventually was successful [3]

---

[3] IVF is a stressful process and involves several steps:
- ovarian stimulation,
- egg retrieval,
- sperm retrieval,
- fertilisation,
- embryo transfer.

A cycle of IVF can take about two to three weeks, and more than one cycle may be required. There are many issues which militate against success with the age of the mother being. an important factor.
A study in 2011 carried out by the NHS showed IVF treatments that resulted in a live birth was:
29% for women under 35
15% for women aged 38 to 39
9% for women aged 40 to 42

She carried him to full term and the birth was vaginal with no complications. The first week after the birth he just slept and fed. His parents were over the moon.
Around a week later Johnny's behaviour changed. He began to cry without apparent reason, sleep became erratic, he couldn't be put down without immediately waking and crying. He hated being picked up by anyone other than his mother. Although he was feeding well, he wasn't thriving emotionally and seemed very unhappy. His parents by then were exhausted from lack of sleep.

When I examined Johnny, he wasn't trusting of me, so I treated him in his mother's arms. During the first session he didn't want to 'acknowledge' me. At best he tolerated my presence, but after a short while began to cry and protest.

What had happened to baby Johnny? From a content baby, asleep for most of the time, he now was hypervigilant, uncomfortable, unhappy, and overwhelmed.

Why the sudden change in his behaviour and why was he so disturbed?

Initially, after the birth, he was sleeping and feeding well. A neonate in their first week mainly just sleeps and wakes for food. Sleeping after the birth is natural and allows the body's energy reserves to restore. However, into his second week he slept less and was more awake when in his mother's arms - a place of relative safety and security. To accommodate other people at this stage was too much for

---

In addition, a pregnancy following IVF treatment slightly increases the chance of pre-eclampsia, growth retardations and bleeding.
https://www.nhs.uk/conditions/ivf/

him to handle. For Johnny to overcome what seemed to be trauma would take time and patience.

The mother constantly expressed guilt of not being able to help her baby. She felt completely inadequate. It was important for her to hear my explanation and approach how to support him. Naturally any explanation needed to be sensitive and respectful towards her feelings. As such my words needed to emphasise that it is understandable that an IVF procedure and subsequent pregnancy would deeply affect her. She expressed her constant fear of a spontaneous miscarriage. She would think and dream about it almost every hour throughout the pregnancy.

It needs to be emphasised that offering craniosacral therapy to support the mother is important, especially as her anxieties were so strong and deeply ingrained. Perhaps these chronic feelings had been 'translated' by the developing baby into a fear of annihilation. Many authors have written about this possibility. [4]

Johnny did not have the 'resources' to resolve these complex emotions. However, his behaviour was not inevitable, as there is much to understand around the topic of the sentient foetus, but it is a possible explanation of Johnny's state.

I thought it would be helpful to connect to his root chakra. The root chakra is the body's most primal energy centre, being located at the base of the spine. Working with this hypothesis I focused on supporting what could be

---

[4] For extensive articles and books about the sentient foetus, see publications by David Chamberlain, Michel Odent, Raymond Castellino, Leah LeGoy and others.

Johnny's fear of dying translated as a general mistrust of others and hypervigilance. He did not at this stage have the ability to relate positively to the world around him.

The root chakra is concerned with the energy associated with instinct, safety, and survival, such as found with the fight or flight response, and can be useful to work with in these special circumstances. A harmonious root chakra will help Johnny to feel grounded and more confident.[5]

I placed my hand under his sacrum, visualising his root chakra, colour red, at the base of his spine. I spoke softly that he was now safe and can begin to trust the world around him; all is now well. After doing this for several minutes he began to relax and kept his gaze directed towards me. I continued with the verbal affirmations for about 10 minutes, after which he wanted to stop.

The outcome was that by the next session Johnny was relating and more tolerant to others. His crying did not cease completely at this stage but significantly improved. He had grown in confidence, felt safer and willing to engage with his surroundings. He would have improved in the fullness of time but, in my view, a craniosacral approach helped considerably to move the process forward.

There is much to commend working with chakras with babies, its incorporation into the craniosacral sessions felt quite natural.

◆◆◆

---

[5] Chakra healing: see: https://www.chakras.info/root-chakra-healing/

Part 3: Case History

Finding out what happened

The baby may be asleep on arrival, in a buggy or being held, allowing the opportunity to gently ask pertinent questions. So much can be learnt about the baby's disposition (and that of the parents) with considered questioning.

How was the pregnancy?
A general question to start proceedings, which allows a wide scope of answers. Was it invitro fertilisation (IVF)?

How long had they been trying?
Due to the high failure rate with IVF, there may be additional emotional investment in their baby, manifesting in over-anxiety and wanting to 'do everything right'.

Previous miscarriages?
This can be a big emotional issue. Both parents, and particularly the mother, may have been in a constant state of vigilance during the pregnancy, especially during the first trimester. The developing foetus may have been affected by the mother's emotional state, which could persist for the duration of the pregnancy.

Any complications during the pregnancy?
For example, gestational diabetes, break-through bleeding, pre-eclampsia.

Any complications during the birth?
How long did it take to become fully dilated? How long was the pushing stage?

Where was the birth, hospital or at home?

Were there signs of the baby's distress?

What was the birth position?

LOA (Left Occiput Anterior) is the most frequent position. LOP (Left Occiput Posterior) face presenting - meaning the mother sees the full face, as the baby emerges from the vagina. LOP generally requires the use of forceps; the mother's peritoneum usually cut to allow easier access. The baby emerging from a LOP position will present with a squashed face due to bony pressure from the mother's pubis. Further pressure on the temporals and orbital region is usually caused by the forceps, leaving pronounced bruising on either side of the face.

It can be very helpful to ask to see photos taken soon after the birth to identify traumatised areas. [6]

---

[6] Face presenting births (LOP) occur in about 1 in 500 full term births.
https://www.open.edu/openlearncreate/mod/oucontent/view.php?id=276&printable=1
See also for extensive information about pregnancy and birth:
https://www.verywellfamily.com/

Observing the Baby: With the baby on the treatment table suggest to the parents to sit back and relax! The purpose of this is for you, the practitioner, to commence bonding with the baby.

The parents may unconsciously 'interfere' with this process by trying to attract the baby's attention, encouraging her to be 'good'. Explanations of craniosacral therapy may be useful to give them permission to 'chill'.

By this time, you will have some idea of the baby's story; essential information to build the beginnings of an empathic relationship, perhaps starting with a verbal welcome with a smile. Throughout this examination the baby may not want to look at you. She may be interested in staring at a light, or somewhere above your head, or on a pattern on your clothes, or find something interesting about the wallpaper, but not at you! Doing so may be too much for her to take in at this stage. No rush, just observe for several minutes, after which a gentle contact can be made, such as a light touch hand to hand. The purpose of this approach is to be non-invasive and respectful.

Contact on the feet or under the sacrum can follow. The practitioner's body language needs to be super-relaxed, well-grounded, and anxiety-free, with facial expressions of wonderment.

In addition to the birth story, further observations can be very revealing, such any asymmetries of the face and cranium. Facial asymmetries tell us where pressure was applied in the birth canal and likewise with body shapes. Look for clues for the discomfort the baby may have experienced during their birth.

The baby's position in the pelvis is generally Left Occiput Anterior (LOA) and the mother's lumbosacral promontory offers a bony obstacle affecting the left side of the baby's body, particularly the face and cranium, which would have been squashed against this part of the pelvis.

The purpose of such detailed observation is to further detail the journey the baby has experienced.

Limb Movements Limbs may offer further clues, such as frantic cycling of legs to relieve abdominal tension or the continuing urge to push themselves out of the birth canal. Movement of arms at first may appear to be random but also can be repetitive. The baby may be trying to draw your attention to a specific area of discomfort, such as to their cranium or abdomen.

Body movements – Is there a patten of unwinding of fascial tissue, such as the head moving from side to side, or a limb moving independently? Such movements are consistent, whereas movement associated with discomfort appear more random and periodic.

Notice the ability to move head left and right. Preference to one side may indicate that the head was pushed to one side for a long period of time. This is assessed with the baby lying down, as she cannot hold her head up at this stage.

Hear how they are crying? They may be upset due to not 'being ready' for the birth, or upset from being stuck in the birth canal, or angry at the whole painful experience, or disturbed because of swallowing meconium [7]

All these aspects are part of their story, which the baby wants us to 'hear' and understand. But the cries of a baby are not always about the past – as the baby may be frightened in that moment and wants to be held for comfort or reassurance, or perhaps they are hungry or just need a change of nappy!

◆◆◆

---

[7] Meconium is a tar-like substance excreted by the baby (in fact, it's their first poo). Babies who are stressed during delivery can pass meconium when they are still in the womb and can inhale it creating serious pulmonary problems.

Part 4:
Continuing the Enquiry

*Look for vital clues
to show what happened*

Manage the Session: It is possible after the baby has arrived at your clinic, she may want a feed followed by a nappy change, and perhaps a top-up feed after that! All of which can eat into the available session time, and this might be as far as you get in the first meeting. Perhaps negotiate with the parent at this stage an extension to the session.

Continue the Examination: Initiate skin to skin contact - gently take her hand in yours. If she wants to move her arm, go with it. The point here is to demonstrate to the baby you are not a threat but offering a gentle benevolent energy. It's important to realise that babies are very sensitive to anxiety energy around them (see Part 5). Hence your touch must be relaxed, respectful and calm. Eventually she will make an inquisitive eye contact.

Let go of the hand and lift the legs to place your hand under the sacrum. The main purpose here is to gently lift the pelvis, which helps the baby to relax as they bring their legs up.
 This is useful if the baby is experiencing abdominal discomfort, wind, colic, and distention. Your free hand can

very gently be placed on the abdomen to bring into your awareness any sensitive areas of the viscera.

Continue to be still in yourself and continue to observe. Several minutes would have now passed and you are still getting to know the baby. She is also getting to know and accept your presence and touch.

Take your hand that was on the abdomen and move it to the cranium, so you are holding the whole central nervous system between your hands.

How does she feel? For example, an energetic sense of compression longitudinally? This would be quite usual if the baby was stuck, during which time there was a prolonged period of uterine pressure on the sacrum, which can translate up the spinal column into the cranium.

Perhaps she feels like a bag of fluid between your hands, indicating she is in a relaxed positive state, or she may feel compartmentalised, possibly along the transverse diaphragms. This could arise if there's localised trauma or restrictions.

Just holding and observing the space between your hands may be enough for the release of induced fulcrums brought about from the pregnancy and birth. There might be a delay period before her body 'lets go' usually by the next day or possibly in that moment.

Now draw your attention to the baby's face and cranium. Recall her birth photos, revealing any sites of bruising and distortions. A more detailed observation is now required. You have already observed the baby but now look carefully and more thoroughly at the face. Examine the temple regions for flatness. Move the head to one side to see the shape of the occiput. Is it asymmetrical or flattened? Look for vital clues to show what happened during the birth.

Where was the pressure felt while she was in the birth canal, where do current discomforts remain? Look at the ears, are they level with each other? If not, this could indicate a functional occipital rotation.

Look at the eyes, are they level and horizontal to the mouth? Generally, being stuck in a LOA position result in a compression of the left-hand side of the face from pressure of being up against the sacral promontory and the left orbital area is often affected (see Figs 1-3).

The mandible, which almost hangs free, is easily pushed to one side or the other. Fortunately, these issues soon resolve themselves, but underlying trauma memory may persist in which case a cranial treatment of gentle holding of the face may be helpful.

When the birth position is LOP 'Face Presenting', this means the mother views the baby's face as it emerges. Often with this position the baby emerges showing a 'battered' appearance having been subjected to direct pressure from the mother's pubis bone (see Fig 4).

An assisted delivery with forceps usually leaves bruised areas where the head and face took the brunt of the pressure. These marks and discomfort may last for some time. Likewise, with a ventouse assisted delivery, the parietal bone on one side can be distorted and sensitive

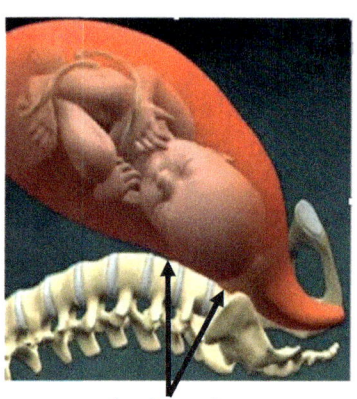

Figure 1: Left Lie Baby pushed against the mother's Lumbosacral Promontory

Lumbosacral Promontory

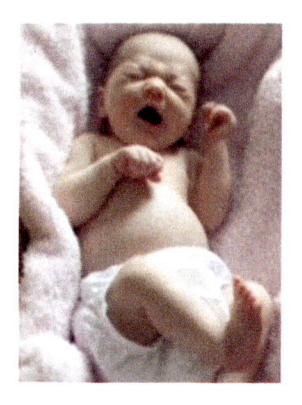

Figure 2: Typical 'Banana' shaped baby arising from pressure along the left-hand side.

26

Figure 3:
Typical Left-Lie Appearance:
Where the left side has been pushed against the mother's Lumbosacral Promontory.

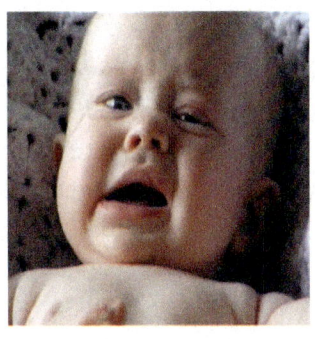

- LHS: Frontal & Temporal areas flatter.

- LHS: orbit smaller, lower & nearer to the nose.

- LHS ear flatter and possibly lower than RHS due to occipital rotation.

- Mandible and nose pushed off-centre towards the RHS

Figure 4:
Face Presenting Baby

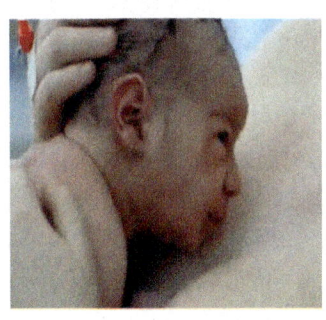

- Typically showing general compression to face and cranium.

- Battered appearance to face.

By the time the baby comes for craniosacral treatment most of the bruising and swelling probably would have diminished. Seeing the photos and hearing what the parents say adds to your knowledge of the baby's story.

Often babies who have had a ventouse extraction detest wearing hats or having their head pushed through clothes. It's no longer painful (but can be), it's more about memory of the discomfort.

It is highly likely that although these emergency measures were necessary and couldn't be avoided at the time, particularly if the baby showed signs of distress or the mother was physically and mentally exhausted, these procedures may not be without pain, trauma, and subsequent discomfort for the baby.

Examine the Palate:
Obtain the permission of the parent and place your cleaned little finger (with a short nail) in the baby's mouth with the pad of the finger pointing towards the upper palate.

Be careful not to place the finger too far back near the soft palate, to avoid the baby's gag reflex.

The purpose is to feel the height of the arch and to assess her power of sucking. The tongue should push hard enough to keep your finger pressed up against the upper palate. If it feels weak suspect a tongue-tie and refer to a local breastfeeding counsellor for confirmation.

It is possible a heightened upper palate may be a consequence of a ventouse extraction and the baby's tongue can't push high enough to form a good latch.

Fortunately, with the majority this is soon resolved by rapid growth, and meanwhile feeding may have to be supplemented with a bottle. All this can take a time to assess.

Craniosacral therapists empathise to provide a therapeutic environment within which healing, and development can occur. 'How are you feeling right now?' is a question that might be asked of a patient - babies are approached with the same curiosity.

Rather than verbalising this, the question is communicated via touch, facial expression and body language while simultaneously offering admiration and affection. She will respond if she feels safe and secure, but it may take a while for her to reach this stage.

The craniosacral therapist's task overall is to sense what the baby is feeling, and be well informed of the pregnancy, birth, and postpartum issues.

A Timeline of Events:
Throughout the session let the parents take you through the events as they see it. This may be the first time they have done this with anyone, and their account may be highly charged. Anger may emerge, directed towards the hospital or individual staff. The wise practitioner should just listen and be sympathetic.

All the knowledge that has been collated about the baby is the foundation that underpins an empathic approach. You 'understand' the baby's trauma, you can now empathise with how they are feeling.
This is further developed in Part 6.

Case Study: Baby Susana:

Sometimes it's not possible to build a comprehensive case-history in the first session, as with baby Susana.

Her mother was not forthcoming regarding details as she was still emotionally processing the birth, which was 2 weeks previously. There had been life threatening complications.

She had no photos to show, as her partner had taken them and hadn't copied them to her yet. I asked if it was possible to bring them to the next session? Her response was indifference. Clearly, the mother was still feeling withdrawn and disassociated from the whole experience.

I offered to treat her as well, with the baby in her arms. Sitting propped up on the treatment table she held Susana, who was asleep, while I placed my hands simultaneously on both.
I held this position for a period. I was focussing on her daughter, looking for clues on the face and cranium. Surprisingly, no obvious clues were visible. In fact, the face and head looked very symmetrical.
I said, 'I'm assuming you had a caesarean', to which she nodded.

She had experienced, I later found out, a prolonged birth where Susana hadn't been progressing well. The amniotic sac ruptured, and the fluids contained meconium (see footnote 7). An emergency caesarean ensued, during which there was a serious haemorrhage.

This was a frightening experience for the mother. In fact, she revealed later she rationally felt she was dying, as the blood loss was considerable. [8]

The full story of Susana's birth was revealed over the next couple of sessions, with incomplete parts and not in any chronological order.

There was no rush; the mother needed time, space, and support to tell the story of her daughter's birth.

◆◆◆

---

[8] Although accountable for only 8% of maternal deaths in developed countries, postpartum haemorrhage is the second leading single cause of maternal mortality, ranking behind preeclampsia/eclampsia. Globally, postpartum haemorrhage is the leading cause of maternal mortality. The condition is responsible for 25% of delivery-associated deaths, and this figure is as high as 60% in some countries.
https://www.medscape.com/answers/796785-122141/

Part 5:
Fish, Babies and The Polyvagal System

The need to feel safe and comfortable

What do fish and babies have in common? Look at a fish and notice on its skin a visible line on each side running laterally down the length of its body from behind the gills to the tail. This is their Lateral Line System. It's a sensory system which constantly monitors the surrounding environment such as movement, temperature, water pressure, sounds and suchlike.

By noticing the environment in this way, the fish finds ideal safe surroundings. The lateral line gives early warning signals of a predator and other adverse conditions that could be threatening. This system is extraordinary and highly sophisticated, and yet it is only the beginning of what will eventually evolve in mammals as part of the vagus, the 10th cranial nerve.

The mammalian vagus enervates much of the viscera, but in addition contains an enhanced version of the lateral line system found in fish. It is believed for babies their polyvagal system is vital for their behavioural and probably also for their cognitive development. The Polyvagal Theory was proposed by Stephen Porges in 1994 and there is much to commend it, suggesting there are two distinct parts, the dorsal and ventral vagal systems.[9]

This concept links the evolution of the mammalian autonomic nervous system to social behaviour. The theory divides the vagus into two parts, namely the dorsal and ventral systems. The dorsal part concerns itself with the functionality of much of the viscera and organs generally below the diaphragm, while the ventral vagal system acts, not unlike an internal lateral line system, interacting with

---

[9] The dorsal branch of the vagal complex (DVC) originates in the dorsal motor nucleus considered by the theory to be the older branch. Polyvagal theory calls this the 'vegetative vagus' because it sees it as being associated with survival strategies such as animals "freezing" when threatened, for example a mouse when attacked by a cat. It controls most of the visceral organs, such as the digestive tract.
The ventral vagal complex (VVC), with increased neural complexity, is said to have evolved in mammals as a more sophisticated system to enrich behavioural and affect responses to an increasingly complex environment.
Polyvagal theory calls this the "smart vagus" because it associates it with the regulation of social behaviour, including social communication and calming strategies.
To maintain homeostasis, the central nervous system responds constantly, via neural feedback, to environmental cues. Stressful events disrupt the rhythmic structure of autonomic states, and subsequently behaviour. The Polyvagal Theory provided us with a more sophisticated understanding of the biology of safety and danger, one based on the subtle interplay between the visceral experiences of our own bodies and the voices and faces of the people around.
It explains why a kind face, or a soothing tone of voice can dramatically alter the way we feel. It helped us understand why attuning with another person can shift us out of disorganized and fearful states. Porges's theory makes us look beyond the effects of fight or flight and put social relationships front and centre in our understanding of trauma. (Wiki)

other cranial nerves. After the birth, a baby only slightly interacts with the world and with those around - sleep and feeding are their priorities in the first week or so.

Slowly, social interactions occur and the baby's own vagal ventral complex, together with other cranial nerves, increasingly react and synchronise with their surroundings.

The function of the ventral vagal system is best explained by observing how a baby interacts:

Carefully observe a new-born when a parent or carer picks them up. What happens?

The baby will look at the parent's face, but they're not just casually looking, this will be an intense stare locked on particularly to the parent's eyes. They are also listening for aural signals.

What is happening in this exchange is the need for them to feel safe and comfortable – confirming that all is well and there's no threat or danger present. Porges suggests the baby is also seeking clues to confirm their sense of self as well as their own safety.

The constant reassurance of facial expressions from the parent, such as a smile, and the quiet gentle tones of their voice, stimulate the baby's vagal complex affecting increased activity of the parasympathetic autonomic nervous system. Consequently, the heart rate reduces, the depth of breathing increases and reduces peristalsis, all resulting in a sense of calmness.

The polyvagal theory suggests this is not learnt behaviour but instinctive - the start of the baby's foundation of social interactional behaviour.

This explanation emphasises why it's valuable in craniosacral work to actively model and offer a sense of safety and reassurance when working with babies, particularly with those that exhibit traumatic behaviour. If a baby is showing signs of trauma, the aim of this approach is to increase parasympathetic activity and consequently reduce the 'flight and fight' hormones, such as adrenaline, which will be circulating in their system.

Sometimes parents may not 'get it right' and give 'unhelpful' signals - they try to 'control' what their baby is feeling by 'shushing' them for example.

In contrast, the practitioner's approach is to encourage the reduction of sympathetic control of the vital organs. This purposely promotes, in the baby, feelings of safety and increases the ability to socially interact with others. This is well demonstrated when the practitioner approaches a baby for the first time. It is not unusual for the baby to initially avoid eye contact but eventually, after a period, will look at the face of the practitioner for reassurance of self.

This stage of development is important and needs to occur before any resolution of her trauma can proceed. The practitioner needs to be patient, as this connection between the baby and the therapist may take time to be established.

Case Study: Baby Rhys

His parents referred to him as a 'super-cool baby'. He engaged with the new surroundings of the treatment room and appeared to be relaxed. In general, he fed and slept well for a month-old baby. Yet all was not as it seemed.
His birth wasn't straightforward. His mother had developed gestational diabetes and was very closely monitored in the last trimester. There was concern the baby would be too large for a vaginal birth, and the mother's sugar levels were jumping about.

Ten days before the due date she had an emergency caesarean. Rhys appeared during the early days to be calm, fed well and happy. Then the reflux started, occurring after every feed. It didn't seem to bother him, and he showed no signs of discomfort such as arching his back or periodic screaming. He remained calm and engaging.

When I came to examine him, he was quiet and remained relaxed. I felt no longitudinal compression - a distinct energetic state that can arise from strong uterine contractions, which I often associate with reflux and colic conditions - but there had been no uterine contractions as this was a caesarean birth.

Throughout he kept his parents in view. I tried to turn his head to engage with me, but he resisted very strongly. I checked his body once more and there was no tension, no obvious panic.

I asked his mother to pick him up as I wanted to carefully observe him again in her arms to determine if there was an issue with his neck. He seemed content and was moving his head freely. I remained curious as to what was causing the reflux. I felt there was something that didn't quite gel with this 'super-cool' baby. He was calm and content and casually looking around. I needed to engage with him while he was in the safe place of his mother's lap.

I laid my hands on his solar plexus and began talking, with soft tones and smiling eyes. His body was already relaxed but I was waiting for a deeper relaxation and an eye-to-eye connection between us. This didn't happen immediately, but after ten minutes I placed him back on the table and there he made eye contact for the first time.

Significantly, his body didn't appear to further relax, but instead a wave of stillness enveloped both of us, as he 'accepted' me. Both of our ventral vagal systems were engaging. I continued offering verbally empathic words concerning the caesarean and the danger of his mother's gestational diabetes. I conveyed with my body, voice, and facial expression he was safe now and much loved.

Later, I heard from the father, Rhys had slept for a few hours afterwards, which was very unusual. A positive response indicating some internalised resolution was taking place.
In the following days, the reflux had virtually stopped, now occurring perhaps only once a day compared to several times previously.

Before I saw Rhys, he had kept his circle of trust to only his parents. Interestingly, outside of this arena his response was not to engage with others, almost in denial that anyone else existed beyond his parents.

It is possible this created an emotional conflict that became translated into a disturbed stomach and reflux; a condition he was prepared to accept, to feel safe and secure. For Rhys feeling safe and secure was his instinctive priority.

◆◆◆

Part 6: Empathy, Love and Attachment Theory

The practitioner's role is to guide and help the baby to 'manage' their emotions.

The craniosacral therapist's empathic approach is different to that of parents as there are no attached preconditions. So, it is important when meeting a mother and baby for the first time to be clear as to the differences between empathy, sympathy, and compassion.

Empathy:
Empathy is feeling what the other is feeling. For example, a person might be grieving for a dead relative and being empathic would mean the listener genuinely feels the pain of the lost relative, experiencing the grieving pains.

To an empathic listener this reaction is not a product of conscious thought but a natural visceral response towards another.

An empathic response also can refer to the whole emotional spectrum, including laughter, happiness, and joy as well as grief, tears and pain.

Empathy is an essential component of craniosacral therapy.

Sympathy:
This refers to understanding what another is feeling and comprehending why they may be feeling this way.

For example, having sympathy towards a person who is grieving for a dead relative is not feeling the same emotions, nor the pain but understanding why and what the other person is feeling.

Strictly speaking sympathy does not represent an emotional attachment towards the one who is suffering.

Compassion:
Compassion is an emotional response to sympathy or empathy and involves the desire to help, to relieve the suffering of the other.

The practitioner consciously wanting to help is not useful in the clinical setting as this can blur professional boundaries. The practitioner's judgement and emotional state will 'get in the way' of the session and reduce the effectiveness of any resolution of the other's suffering.

On meeting a baby for the first time they can be in a state of emotional confusion and unable to 'process' what has happened or what is happening. The practitioner's role is to guide and help the baby to 'manage' their emotions.

We show the baby that we 'understand' what they have experienced and 'hear' their cries. The practitioner is aware, from observations and the case-history, what has happened. A knowledge of the events allows the practitioner to display empathic feelings and gestures.

One must be genuine - there is no place for a learned protocol. One can't be genuine unless it comes from the heart, from a deep empathic place.

Feelings of safety, security, being cared for and unconditional love create intense feelings of well-being and happiness.

Physiologically what occurs within the baby's and practitioner's bodies is a state of 'love', leading to trust and relaxation involving an increased activation of their mutual vagal systems.

Love:

Love in craniosacral practice is more than a mutual physiological response as it provides support to process feelings and move on.

Babies can 'control' their feelings but only up to a point. Their inexperience with their emotions and reactions to the outside world can quickly become overwhelming. Staring at a baby, for example, may be too intense for the baby to 'process'.

Love has a powerful impact on the development and 'Attachment Theory' offers an approach which can be beneficial to the baby. [10]

Attachment Theory:

Although love can be described as just a feeling, a 'nice warm feeling towards another' - it's also about how you support the other person. We do this by being

---

[10] Attachment theory: British psychologist John Bowlby was the first attachment theorist. He described attachment as a "lasting psychological connectedness between human beings."
Some of the earliest behavioural theories suggested that attachment was simply a learned behaviour. These theories proposed that attachment was merely the result of the feeding relationship between the child and the caregiver. Because the caregiver feeds the child and provides nourishment, the child becomes attached. Bowlby observed that feedings did not diminish separation anxiety. Instead, he found that attachment was characterised by clear behavioural and motivation patterns. When children are frightened, they seek their primary caregiver in order to receive both comfort and care. Attachment, the theory suggests, is innate and essentially supports the safety and survival of the baby. (Wiki)

empathic and understanding about what they're feeling, noticing their body language, non-verbal signals and responding to it all. Parents instinctively give feedback continuously with facial gestures. These gestures reflect to the baby what kind of state they are in.

Keenly watch a parent's facial expressions in response to their baby that show their baby's feelings are 'understood'.

This 'mirroring back' instinctively conveys to the baby the sense that they have been 'heard'.
The parent may add to this by offering a reassuring expression, such as a nod of the head. All these interactions are subtle and quickly happen and are generally repeated over a period.

The craniosacral therapist's empathic approach is similar to that of the parents, in 'mirroring' to the baby, but different, as there are no attached preconditions. The practitioner can offer what is required by the baby to move on from their traumatic birth.

This is a fundamental point, as babies cannot 'manage' their emotions, and in the therapeutic context the practitioner endeavours to model this with them. The practitioner models this, like the parent, through facial expressions and behaviour, mainly by smiling, gentle eye contact and relaxed body language. In addition, the gentle touch of holding their hands and a soft calming voice further encourages the baby's own feelings of love and safety.

Attachment theory teaches us to reflect to the baby what we observe and feel its significance. A baby learns about themselves through our body language. Importantly, the baby's sense of self is enhanced with these gestures.

This interaction between the practitioner or paren't and the baby goes back and forth. This supporting and affectionate behaviour stimulates the release of oxytocin (the 'love' hormone) to flow from the baby's hypothalamus into their bloodstream. In fact, it is a mutual response experienced by both the practitioner and the baby, as feelings of love, contentment and trust emerge. The baby's sense of self is enhanced as the practitioner in that moment becomes their 'best friend'.

Babies do not develop a strong sense of self without this interaction and feedback from others. Furthermore, it has been suggested that oxytocin may play an important role in the development of parts of the brain concerned with social behaviour [11]

For example, as babies are sentient beings, they can present as being 'stuck' in their traumatic experience,

---

[11] Role of Oxytocin in the neonatal brain: see Kent State University 2018: https://www.kent.edu/research/kent-state-research-review-2019/news/exploring-oxytocins-role-developing-brain

unable to move on. This may occur if the baby had difficulty in navigating the birth canal. They may be reliving this by continuously turning their head to find a way through (see case study below).

What is offered by the practitioner is totally unconditional. In contrast, parents will often react to their baby's distress by trying to soothe them.

The practitioner's role is to show the baby and the parents a different response. 'Shushing' the baby may be needed, but without the mirroring aspect of empathic interacting, the baby's anguish may be prolonged.

The practitioner can offer expressions of delight, unconditional love, supported by a subtle touch of the hands on the baby's body, which convey that all is now safe and well.

Observing a mother with her baby shows she does this instinctively, but practitioners do this with 'purpose'.

The practitioner's interaction with the baby may be sufficient to help the baby to emotionally move on, but the response from the baby is unpredictable and may require repeated efforts to achieve this.

Naturally, the role of the parents is crucial in the baby's emotional development. The practitioner can model this interaction for the parents, and they will learn from watching and listening.

This empathic approach encourages healing and acceptance, and is often accompanied by short periods of stillness, which may come and go throughout the craniosacral session.

Case Study: Baby Asha

Asha's father came to see me when she was two months old. He was worried as he felt something was 'wrong'. She would not allow anyone other than her parents to hold her, otherwise she would loudly cry and scream. Asha now and then would also cry inconsolably in their arms.

They have visited their GP, who referred Asha to a neonatal paediatrician, but neither offered an explanation.

Asha's history showed she had a difficult and prolonged birth. After several hours of labour Asha was not progressing and her heart rate during contractions was dropping fast and was slow to recover. Eventually the medical team decided to perform an emergency caesarean as she was probably in distress.

This proceeded without complications. I had in mind to gradually approach Asha and initially just sit with her. When Asha was placed on the treatment table she immediately began to scream. She was thrashing her head from side to side. This action didn't stop. She wasn't in pain or discomfort as she stopped crying as soon as she was back in her father's arms, a place of safety.

From the case history the head movements suggested this was her behaviour during the birth - determined to find a passage through the pelvis. Her head, it seemed, wouldn't position itself properly and turning her head from side to side was all she could achieve. This was a frightening and life-threatening experience.

At first, she was held on her father's lap, and I sat close by and waited for her to stop crying. I wanted to reassure her that all was safe and well, but she wouldn't 'acknowledge' my presence and her crying intensified when I lightly laid my hands on her. I wanted another approach.

To resolve her trauma Asha needed to revisit her birth and this time 'get it right'. I placed her on my lap and held her upside down against my legs. She immediately began screaming and rapidly moving her head from side to side. I slowly opened my legs to allow her head to poke through – offering her to re-enact her experience passing through the pelvis.

I explained to the father what I was doing and then the session ran out of time. I suggested to him to try something similar with Asha at home.

The following week Asha came again with her father. He reported they had tried a re-enactment a couple of times. Asha now seemed a little calmer, but he suggested this was probably wishful thinking!
I repeated the 'mock-birth' and although Asha was crying it was less intense than the previous week. She was turning her head from side to side but there were also moments when this stopped.

I tried this again and she cried for just a short period. Also, the head movements were less often and less vigorous. I placed her on the treatment table and although initially there was some crying it was significantly reduced and followed by periods when she was quiet and still.

She would turn her head from time to time towards her father just to check he was there. She also importantly acknowledged my presence.

I place a hand on her and spoke softly offering words of 'understanding'. I held her hand and engaged with her solar plexus. Full of admiration knowing what she had been through I kept mirroring back what I felt in my body of how horrific her experience must have been.

I nodded my head while conveying that she was now safe and well by smiling and looking at her admiringly.

Several minutes passed and I noticed how relaxed she had become. She was in a state of stillness and went into a much-needed sleep. I saw her once more, with her looking at me intently for long periods. I took advantage of the moment and repeated the mirroring of her feelings as well as nodding and smiling, my overall approach was like the previous session

Asha by then had made very good progress and was moving on from her initial trauma. In this interchange she demonstrated her new-found trust in others that went beyond her parents. She was developing a sense of self and engaging with her surroundings.

Asha felt safe at last.

◆◆◆

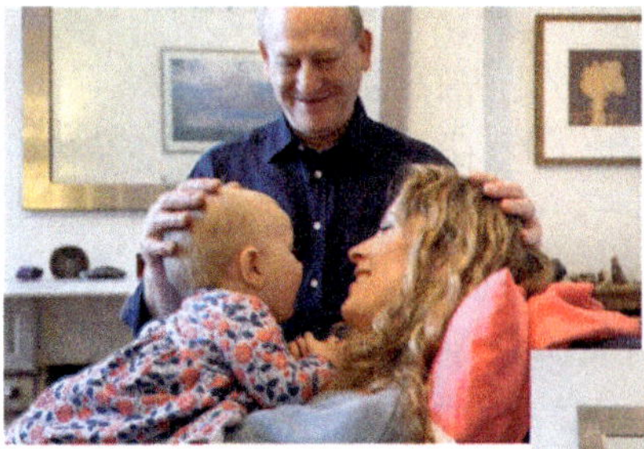

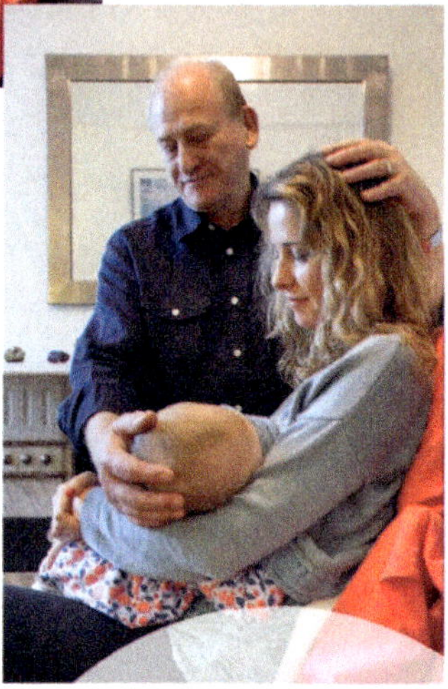

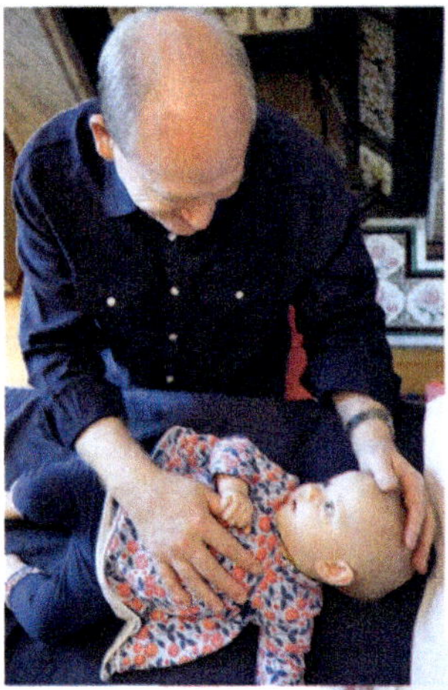

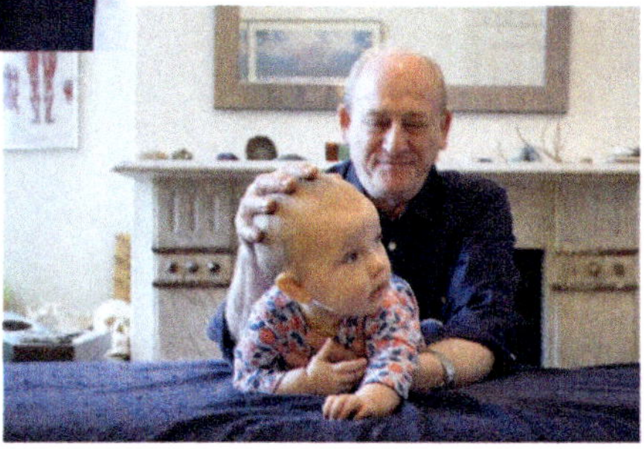

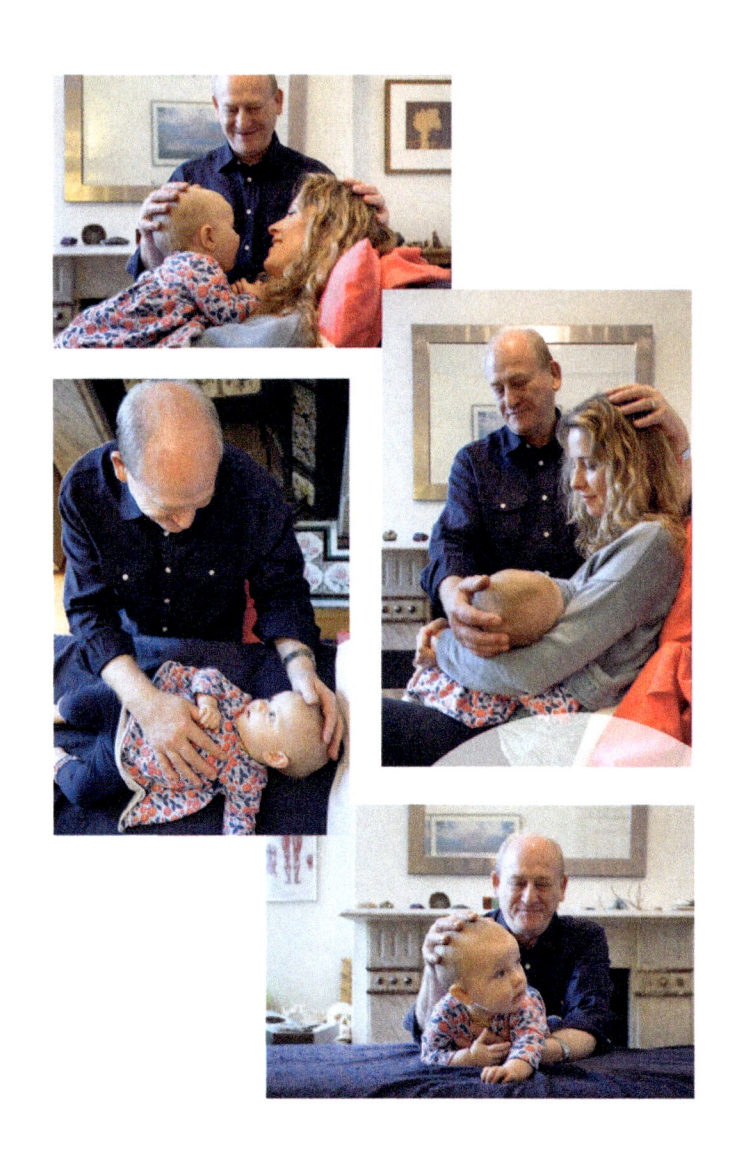

Part 7: Stillness

By dissolving the barriers, fears, and brick walls the baby can let go

In the previous chapter, we have learnt that an empathic approach to babies involves learning, understanding and feeling their experiences they had in the womb, and during the birth. This is one vital aspect of working successfully with babies.

Another essential aspect is being aware of stillness. Stillness constantly arises during craniosacral sessions. It may last for just a few seconds or a few minutes. This is nothing new to a craniosacral practitioners, as out of stillness the therapeutic process develops and is indicative that emotional resolution, or re-organisation of tissue, is occurring. A positive state to experience.

By dissolving the barriers, fears and brick walls the baby can let go, relax and begin to resolve their anxieties.

Case history: Baby Anna

Baby Anna had a difficult birth. She became distressed as her passage through the birth canal was not proceeding well. The mother was fully dilated, but Anna was a large baby and was having difficulty navigating the pelvis. However, the baby's distress lessened and so the midwife decided to let things proceed naturally, which they did, albeit slowly.

Later, Anna displayed distress again, she was crowning with each contraction but not moving her body further. The medical team decided to use forceps, which was successful in pulling her out.

The parents reported Anna seemed angry when emerging into daylight; this wasn't surprising considering the discomfort offered by the huge forceps clasping her face, frontals and temporal bones. The pressure must have been considerable. She was probably angry at the shock of the final part of the birth and objected to the pain.

After a few days of only sleeping and feeding, Anna became agitated and disturbed. This occurred at various times and wasn't fixed to a particular time of day, but it was happening every day. In her own way she seemed to be revisiting the trauma and trying to process it. She needed help to do so.

On examination she seemed tense and not trusting of me. I just watched her. What was she doing with her limbs? Her legs and arms were flailing about and there wasn't any obvious reason. She wasn't crying but neither was she happy nor even acknowledging my presence. I took hold of her hand and asked her to 'show' me where it hurt? No response from her.

She kept flailing her arms about, but every now and then her free hand would go to her head about the temporal area. I 'asked' her again if that was where it hurt? After a while her movements became less frantic, and I made deeper contact by placing my hand under her sacrum. In that hand I was able also to hold her legs up to reduce tension in her abdomen. (Having a large hand was useful here!). Anna's movements slowed down and eventually came to a stop.

She seemed to be sleepy but remained awake. This stage took about twenty minutes. She was entering into a period of stillness. Her whole body became relaxed, and I looked up at the parents, who both expressed amazement. They hadn't seen their baby before so peaceful while awake.

Together Anna and I remained in this state for several more minutes. I still had her hand in mine and through this touch and expressions conveyed my feelings for her, conveying my understanding of the hurt and distress of her delivery. In those few minutes, with the empathy she was receiving, she came to 'let go' and to begin to emotionally move on.

Her parents told me a few days later how well she slept that night and significantly she had only a few short periods of agitation subsequently in the following days.

Case History: Baby Tam

Baby Tam came into the treatment room crying and screaming, very upset - her mother was embarrassed and naturally at the end of her tether. Tam didn't want to be fed in that moment and didn't want to be in a strange room with a strange person.

I sat down away from them both. I invited the mother also to sit down with her baby and asked her quietly to tell me about Tam.

Tam was five weeks old. She was upset during the day and into the evening. Eventually she stops crying from exhaustion and then generally sleeps soundly for up to seven hours.

What is significant here is that during her pregnancy the mother had developed gestational diabetes. She became very worried once she knew the cause of her tiredness and thirst. Subsequently, her perusal of the internet scared her; suggesting possibilities of neural defects in her baby, deformed buccal cavity, renal complications and heart defects which can occur with this condition.

Due to her health, she was induced at 39 weeks. Contractions commenced and continued for 5-6 hours, during which Tam's heart rate kept dipping.

When born, Tam needed oxygen, although she was not blue, but the cord was wrapped around her neck and initially she was having difficulty breathing. Fortunately, this persisted for only a short period.

Her first week was 'good', reported her mother. Then the daytime screaming started - accompanied with long bouts of vigorous hiccups. The mother felt the hiccups were painful for Tam and this was contributing to the screaming.

I put her mind to rest as hiccups in babies look dramatic and troublesome but generally they cause little bother to the baby.

What was significant however was the fearful state the mother experienced during the pregnancy. She was beside herself with worry, realising her baby may suffer ill-effects from the gestational diabetes. Irrationally she felt so guilty.

Her baby, certainly in the latter stages of the pregnancy, was probably aware of the effects of increased adrenaline in the blood stream - increasing heart rate and a heightened state of alertness. The cord around her neck added to the sympathetic stimulation involving pressure on the superior cervical ganglion. It was a very difficult time for them both.

On examination, which wasn't easy as Tam was not trusting the world around her, I projected empathy to her, through my minimal touch, voice and facial expressions. I understood how difficult the pregnancy was for them both. I was conveying an appreciation of how scary and life-threatening this must have been. I 'offered' that all was well now, and she could begin to let go of this experience and move on.

Inducing a birth led to very strong contractions in a relatively short time. This is often translated into a palpable feeling of compression between the thorax and abdomen due to the immense pressure projecting the baby through the birth canal. The stomach in this scenario is often compromised giving rise to acid reflux, irritating the oesophagus as it passes through the diaphragmatic muscle, hence the hiccups.

Tam entered a period of stillness - her agitation lessened but didn't entirely disappear. I felt her stillness lasted for about a minute.

After the initial session the mother reported Tam had been calm, still occasionally upset but significantly less. At the second session, a week later, the same empathic approach was adopted. On this occasion she was accepting of my touch, but there were no further periods of stillness.

The mother reported later that Tam screamed once again for a very short period that night and then it stopped entirely. It seemed 60 seconds of stillness was enough for Tam to kickstart the process of resolving her trauma.

◆◆◆

Part 8: Feeding & Tongue-Tie

Resolution of the baby's or mother's trauma will be delayed if feeding is problematic.

A consideration of breast feeding is included here as so much depends on getting it right. If feeding is difficult then both the baby and the mother suffer. The baby will be frustrated, hungry and inconsolable. The mother could develop a breast infection, feel emotionally drained and physically exhausted.

The important point here is that any resolution of the baby's or mother's trauma will be delayed if feeding is problematic. Breast feeding depends on an adequate supply of milk and the baby's ability to latch on to the breast efficiently.

The mother's supply may be inadequate at first. This is a normal situation as it will increase with demand. However, if a lip or tongue-tie is present, this may not happen as breast feeding becomes increasingly difficult for both mother and baby.

The baby's mouth needs to be examined by a breastfeeding consultant for tongue/lip ties (see Fig 5). [12]

Figure 5:
Tongue-Tie: The tongue has restricted movement due to the shortness of the Frenulum membrane, which connects the tongue to the floor of the mouth. When feeding is troublesome the Frenulum is commonly divided.

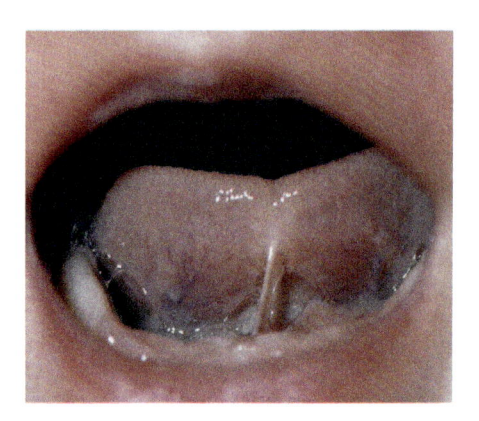

Tongue or lip ties prevent a good latch. Anything less will not create the appropriate flow of milk and eventually place undue wear on the nipples making feeding painful for the mother. This can lead to mastitis, an infection of the milk ducts. Nipple shields can help to prevent this, but babies may not take to breast feeding via a plastic attachment.

Some doctors may not appreciate the difficulty tongue/lip-ties present and assume that in the fullness of time matters

---

[12] Tongue-tie (ankyloglossia): https://www.nhs.uk/conditions/tongue-tie/

will improve. This may be so, but meanwhile mother and baby may be struggling.

When cutting the tongue-tie is performed the improvements to feeding can be dramatic. Despite snipping the tongue-tie, a poor supply of milk or persistence of poor feeding habits, will predict ongoing difficulties. The mother must now resort to using or topping up feeds with formula milk. This can create strong feelings of a 'failed mother', especially as breastfeeding is described as one of the joys of having a baby.

A baby who is a poor feeder may evoke concerns in the mother that there is something wrong with her mothering, or her baby, or both. The mother's state of sleep deprivation may further increase these feelings of inadequacy and helplessness.

Anyone offering advice should be sensitive to these concerns. Obviously, there is much literature to support the advantages of breastfeeding, not only from the uniqueness of the process to the enjoyment of skin-to-skin bonding, but also giving full nutrition to her baby, which importantly begins to establish the baby's gut microbiome.

Also, breast feeding is valuable for digestion and general state of heath. These aspects are vital for optimal health of the baby and should always be kept in mind, which normally it is, by health-visitors, doctors, and breast-feeding counsellors alike. However, breast-feeding often doesn't work out for the mother and baby, and this needs sensitive support from practitioners in general.

Case Study: Brenda

Brenda spent what must be at least 10 hours a day feeding her daughter. Breast feeding was followed by a bottle of expressed milk, which previously had been pumpedfrom the breast. But often the feed had to be topped up with formula.

Brenda was in a constant state of feeling engulfed and wondered if the pump was working efficiently, or whether the tongue-tie had come back? She tried various herbal remedies, essential oils, eating a good diet and remaining well hydrated. She felt she had done everything possible and began to resent the attitudes towards her.
Family and friends would say:
'Breastfeeding is natural, be patient!' or
'Stop moaning and get on with it!'.

She sought craniosacral therapy hoping to reduce her anxiety She had become totally preoccupied with breastfeeding, thinking about it all the time, day and night. The worry increased her tension, anxiety, feelings of uselessness and being an inadequate mother. She began to begrudge her daughter and wasn't enjoying her. But she carried on regardless despite no upturn of the milk production.

At this stage she came to craniosacral therapy hoping it would help. It helped her, but not physiologically. It supported her to arrive at an unexpected decision of acceptance. She stopped trying to breastfeed.

At first the sense of guilt dramatically increased - she felt she had let her daughter down. A few weeks later, at a further session she was feeding exclusively by formula. The important point to note was that they were both so happy! Her daughter was now well fed, putting on weight, sleeping well and content.

Brenda had no misgivings with giving up breastfeeding. She was now looking after her daughter in the best way she could.

Following the craniosacral sessions, she accepted completely she couldn't breastfeed and understood she had no control with this matter. But importantly she knew that she was a good mother in finding a solution.

How does the topic of 'Breast verses Bottle' fit into a craniosacral approach to working with a baby's trauma?
Why is this topic so important in the context of supporting a baby's experience in their early life?

The answer may seem obvious: a well-fed baby is a precondition for a contented and happy baby. But within this scenario, often neglected by professionals, is the mental state of health of the mother, who is expected to just 'get on with the job'.

The feelings of being an inadequate mother are very real and are not easily pushed to one side. Bonding with her baby may well be delayed and her capacity to enjoy her baby could be stilted.

Her ability to provide feedback to her baby, such as 'all is well', will be limited due to her own internal feelings of a 'failed mother'.

For a baby to overcome their internal terrors the relationship with the mother is paramount. The practitioner must be aware of these dynamics as they will affect the ability of the mother to give meaningful and adequate feedback to her child. The therapist's sensitivity to these possibilities is fundamental to any successful consultation.

◆◆◆

Part 9:
New Parents Look After Yourselves

Reassurance is essential

It's valuable to accept there's always an element of trauma for mother and baby. This cannot be said often enough, particularly when new parents seek craniosacral support for themselves and their babies and are usually in a state of turmoil. The world's horizons have narrowed so much they can't see beyond themselves and their baby. They need reassurance, sleep and even more sleep!

Naturally they want their baby to be healthy and happy, feeding to be a joy, sleeping well and completely content. Unfortunately, rarely do these factors all come together, even less so if the birth was traumatic, as it usually is to some degree.

It's useful for parents to realise there's always an element of trauma, whether the birth was vaginal, c-section or no obvious complications at the time. Ante-natal classes tend to emphasise ideal births but assisted births will occur in about 1 in 8 (12%) of births in the UK. About 8 percent of all pregnancies involve complications that, if left untreated, may harm the mother or the baby [13]

A new parent may say to the practitioner,
'What's wrong with my baby?',
'I didn't feel prepared',
'I haven't had time to process what exactly happened',
'I'm so tired'.

Reassurance is essential, which should be forthcoming. In the long-term parents need to be aware of local support structures, such as post-natal groups, local National Birthcare Trust (NCT) groups, breastfeeding consultants, talking therapies, homeopaths, and suchlike.

A baby, who is a poor sleeper, waking several times in the night can be exhausting to care for (and naturally more so for a single parent). Although hard at first, these hurdles are not forever and after 12 weeks most issues would have settled.

In addition, the mother may be recovering from the trauma of the birth, possibly including surgery. Consequently, her bonding with her baby may be delayed or limited. Family and friends are focussed on the baby, but the mother has also been through the birth and needs time and space to reconcile what has happened.

---

[13] Approximately 8% of all pregnancies involve complications: https://www.hopkinsmedicine.org/health/conditions-and-diseases/staying-healthy-during-pregnancy/4-common-pregnancy-complications#:~:text=Most%20pregnancies%20progress%20without%20incident,occur%20unexpectedly%20and%20are%20unavoidable.

Her maternal instincts may be held in abeyance for an undefined period. In most cases, there's no need to pathologise this as post-natal depression (PND), as it can be a natural response, allowing the mother time and space to process her own trauma. However, in a few cases PND may develop into a chronic state, which should be medically assessed.

During any period of mother's withdrawal, her baby may feel confused due to a lack of emotional support, but generally this will be a relatively short period. During this stage super-loving validation from her partner and friends is vital. It is important for themselves and their baby's well-being that parents look after each other and maintain a sense of humour.

Not easy to achieve, not easy at all. When in the dead of night their partner is getting a few hours of quality rest, a parent is woken up to the sound of their baby crying and possibly screaming. The semi-awake parent feels hopelessly inadequate, completely responsible, very tired, cold, and just wants to crawl back into bed!

At a personal level, never has their trust and liking for their partners been under such strain. Sadly, we all know of relationships breaking under these circumstances. So many new parents are inadequately prepared to cope at this stage. Fortunately, patterns and routines get established. But more needs to be done.

New parents need to find a time, even only for a few minutes each day to be together creating a mutual space. This could be a long hug, holding hands for a period, affirmations or an expression of love and gratitude to the other. Offering this advice works wonders, not only for the couple but importantly has a positive effect on the baby.

Their jobs as parents are difficult enough, but they must be mentally and physically in a good place to support their baby's need to overcome any residual birth trauma.

Case Study: Tom and Louise

This couple came to see me with a concern that all was not well with their baby. There were no specific symptoms, but both sought my opinion.

Their baby was 3 months old and on examination nothing significant was found.

What directed me to be concerned was the state of Tom and Louise. Their overall weariness and exhaustion were obvious. The baby wasn't the best of sleepers nor had a good latch, so feeding was an issue causing much discomfort to the mother. But neither was able to organise a long sleep for themselves and even when they occasionally did so, their sleep was light, instinctively keeping an ear open for their baby.

But what drew my attention was the verbal interchange between the parents. It had an edge, a tone which reflected their tiredness and irritation. They were losing mutual respect and love for each other, to the effect I was expecting an explosive argument to develop in front of me around a trivial matter.

I offered a long-term view of what to expect in the coming months, emphasising there was a need to provide support to each other and to arrange support from others; and importantly to keep a sense of humour.

I referred Louise to a breast-feeding counsellor and recommended a couple-therapist. I heard from Louise few months later. Her and Tom were very happy and enjoying their baby, who was in good health sleeping and feeding well.

They had found the therapist immensely helpful; providing the motivation once more to lovingly reconnect with each other and to their baby.

◆◆◆

Part 10:
Giving & Receiving From the Community

The clinic had placed craniosacral therapy in the locality as a vital resource for parents and their babies.

The richest moments in life, I would argue, are when we realise we have achieved something special, which has benefited many others.

I'm not meaning a lottery win, which I then bestow amongst friends and neighbours, but the establishment of a weekly drop-in craniosacral clinic, where over a period of twenty-plus years saw scores of babies, together with their parents and siblings, receiving short low-cost sessions.

The clinic had a slow start in a local community centre. I prepared a leaflet targeting babies and children from a pre-school group, who also used the premises.

Probably out of curiosity, a local health visitor attended the clinic and soon afterwards was recommending it to new mums and dads. She kindly also invited me to her fathers and babies' group, and on several occasions, I offered impromptu sessions to the babies and occasionally to the dads.

The outcome of these initiatives was the clinic was soon busy, each week seeing half a dozen people in the three-hour period.

On arrival at the Community Centre, it was not unusual for me to be greeted by a small queue waiting to put their names on the appointment time sheet.

Meanwhile, the management committee of the centre praised the clinic, as it brought people in touch with other activities in the centre.

After the first year of opening, I contacted new craniosacral graduates inviting them to assist at the clinic and simultaneously gain vital experience, especially working with babies.

Within months the demand for a place to assist was strong. Those attending were usually asked to return to consolidate their experience.

Seeing new babies most weeks meant I could call upon a large pool of parents, who later I would invite to attend a free craniosacral session with their babies held during my advanced courses for craniosacral therapists.

I ran these weekend courses for 10 years, the topic always being 'Baby Trauma'. During each course the therapist participants had the opportunity to work with a baby under my supervision and these events were highly successful and enjoyed by all.

Over the years, hundreds attended the clinic based on its reputation, which went beyond the confines of my immediate locality.

Referrals to my practice and the clinic have been by a variety of professionals, including health visitors, breast-feeding counsellors, senior nurses, general practitioners, and those specialising with tongue-tie division.

The clinic had placed in the locality craniosacral therapy as a vital resource for parents and their babies.
In addition, the clinic importantly enhanced my practice, where I could develop my work more deeply with babies.

Local social media also made a significant difference. When I started to practice, social media was not prominent, but in recent years has blossomed and become a valuable reference place for parents. I have been frequently told that parents heard about craniosacral therapy and the clinic from numerous endorsements found on local social media groups.

Out of curiosity I asked a new mother how she had heard about me and craniosacral therapy?
Her referral came from an unexpected source:

Mary's story:
Following the last pandemic lock-down Mary was desperate to get her hair done. It had been a long time since she was able to get to a hairdresser, not only due to the lockdown but because she was pregnant. Naturally getting about in the latter stages of pregnancy was difficult.

She did eventually get to the hairdresser when her baby was three weeks old, as she wanted to celebrate the event and felt she deserved it!

Her conversation with the hairdresser was the usual chatter, but of course she mentioned her baby and said how difficult the last three weeks had been for herself and partner. She hadn't expected caring for a baby was such hard work.

'How come', said the hairdresser.
'What's been happening?'

She explained her baby was very unsettled, sleeping was erratic, and he didn't seem to be enjoying life. Out of worry, she took him to her GP, who reassured that nothing was wrong. But the doctor's words didn't help.

Hairdresser: 'A year ago, I had a baby girl and a similar situation. She was easily disturbed, very light sleeper and wouldn't sleep for more than an hour at a time.'

'She was very clingy and woke several times in the night. Comfort feeding only slightly helped. My husband and I were at our wits end with worry. We were desperate for a good night's rest. '

'Looking after a baby was a job we weren't prepared for. Our main concerns were the pregnancy and birth. We hadn't given much thought to what would happen after that.'

'Fortunately, a good friend recommended 'cranio' and mentioned a donation based local clinic run by Richard Kramer.'

Two women nearby in the salon sat up and said they knew about this clinic and had taken their babies there! They agreed the 'cranio' sessions had really helped their babies to become settled and sleep well.

'So' said Mary with a smile, in response to my original question,
'That's how I know about you - from my hairdresser'.

I have since retired from the Drop-in Clinic but have left it in the capable hands of two of my colleagues, namely Maria Esposito RCST and Zoe Rigby RCST. They have worked with me for many years, and I am grateful for their devotion to the clinic and to its ethos.

◆◆◆

About The Author

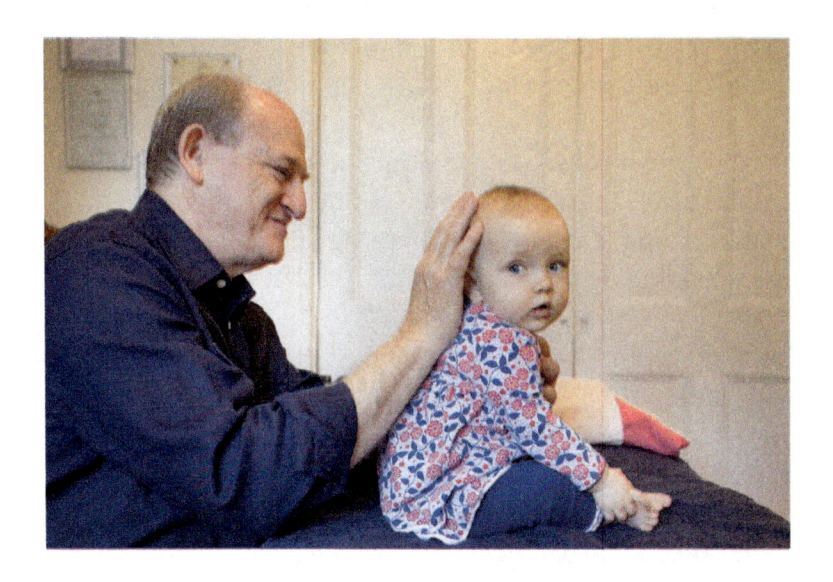

Richard Kramer describes his journey to craniosacral therapy akin to a slow zig-zag dance.

After qualifying as a pharmacologist, he worked in the NHS researching migraine, epilepsy, and muscular dystrophy. He loved the work but felt challenged by the over-dependence on drugs within clinical practice. During this period, he was drawn towards complementary medicine -

emphasising as it does the body's capability to naturally self-heal.

He left the NHS and retrained as a teacher becoming a biology lecturer in further education.
About this time in the early 1990s, based on a friend's recommendation, he recalls taking his son to a craniosacral therapist. He was impressed by the outcome and started to consider a change of direction closer towards complimentary medicine.

In 1997, he enrolled on a diploma course at the College of Craniosacral Therapy in London and on graduating was invited to join the college where he remained for several years, ending up as senior tutor.

During this time, he built a thriving practice in North London and established a weekly drop-in clinic, which was donation-based, offering craniosacral to all, but prioritising babies.
Over the course of more than twenty years scores of people from the locality attended the clinic. Also, many craniosacral graduates sought work-shadowing and assisted under his supervision. The clinic developed a good reputation and was usually oversubscribed.
During this period, he ran several postgraduate craniosacral courses focusing on the many aspects of baby trauma.

Throughout the 2000s he was the Registrar for the Craniosacral Therapy Association (CSTA) and sat on its national committee for 15 years. He was awarded a Fellowship for his services.

Richard continues to live and practice in Crouch End, North London and looks forward to your comments about this book.

He can be contacted at: *mail@richardkramer.co.uk*

◆◆◆

Printed in Great Britain
by Amazon